This Book Belongs To:

....

....

....

Emergency Contacts

Type One Teen

Shot Location

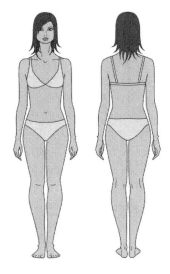 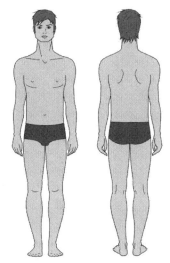

Notes

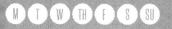

Date: /   /

	Time	Blood Sugar	Carbs	Insulin	Notes
Breakfast					
Snack					
Lunch					
Snack					
Dinner					
Bedtime					
Night					

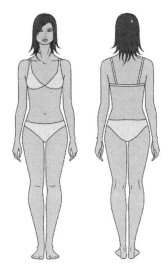

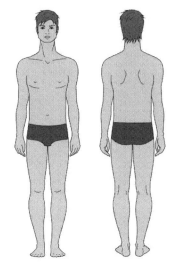

Shot Location

Notes

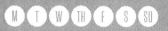

Date: / /

	Time	Blood Sugar	Carbs	Insulin	Notes
Breakfast					
Snack					
Lunch					
Snack					
Dinner					
Bedtime					
Night					

Shot Location

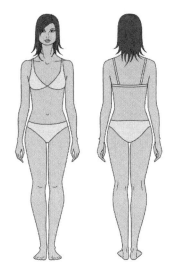 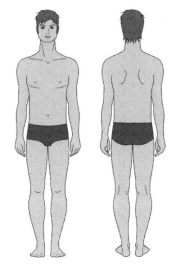

Notes

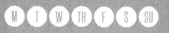
	Time	Blood Sugar	Carbs	Insulin	Notes
Breakfast					
Snack					
Lunch					
Snack					
Dinner					
Bedtime					
Night					

Shot Location

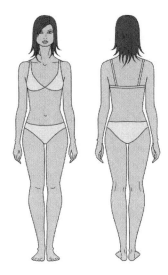
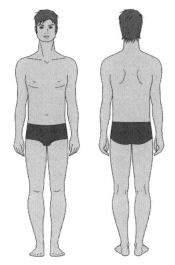

Notes

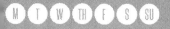

	Time	Blood Sugar	Carbs	Insulin	Notes
Breakfast					
Snack					
Lunch					
Snack					
Dinner					
Bedtime					
Night					

Shot Location

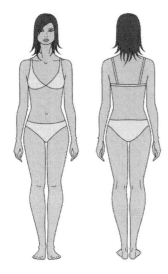

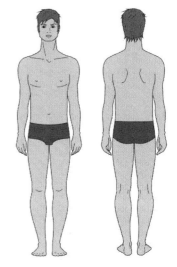

Notes

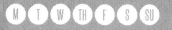

	Time	Blood Sugar	Carbs	Insulin	Notes
Breakfast					
Snack					
Lunch					
Snack					
Dinner					
Bedtime					
Night					

Date: / /

Shot Location

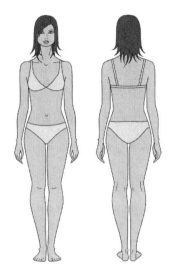

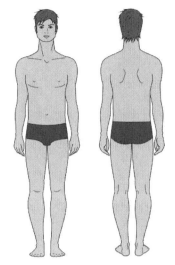

Notes

M T W TH F S SU

Date: / /

	Time	Blood Sugar	Carbs	Insulin	Notes
Breakfast					
Snack					
Lunch					
Snack					
Dinner					
Bedtime					
Night					

Shot Location

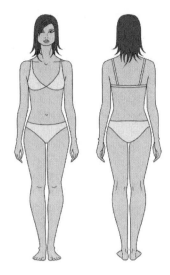

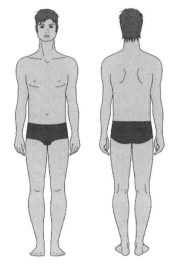

Notes

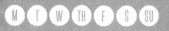
	Time	Blood Sugar	Carbs	Insulin	Notes
Breakfast					
Snack					
Lunch					
Snack					
Dinner					
Bedtime					
Night					

Shot Location

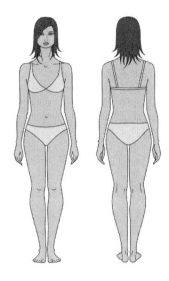 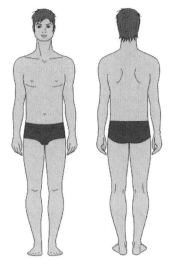

Notes

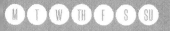
	Time	Blood Sugar	Carbs	Insulin	Notes
Breakfast					
Snack					
Lunch					
Snack					
Dinner					
Bedtime					
Night					

Shot Location

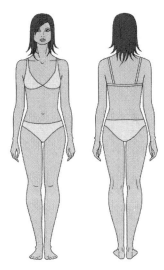

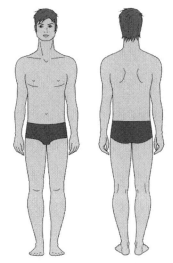

Notes

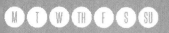

	Time	Blood Sugar	Carbs	Insulin	Notes
Breakfast					
Snack					
Lunch					
Snack					
Dinner					
Bedtime					
Night					

Shot Location

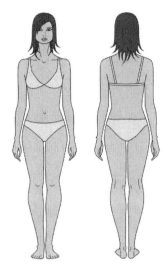 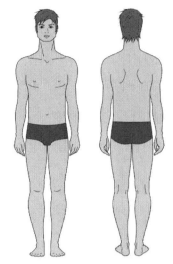

Notes

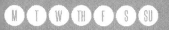

	Time	Blood Sugar	Carbs	Insulin	Notes
Breakfast					
Snack					
Lunch					
Snack					
Dinner					
Bedtime					
Night					

Shot Location

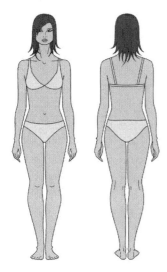
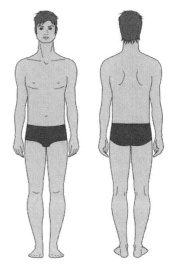

Notes

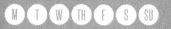
	Time	Blood Sugar	Carbs	Insulin	Notes
Breakfast					
Snack					
Lunch					
Snack					
Dinner					
Bedtime					
Night					

Shot Location

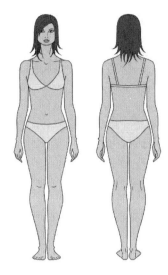

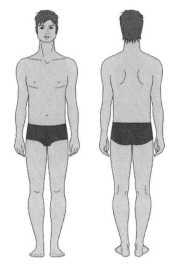

Notes

	Time	Blood Sugar	Carbs	Insulin	Notes
Breakfast					
Snack					
Lunch					
Snack					
Dinner					
Bedtime					
Night					

Shot Location

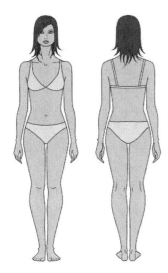
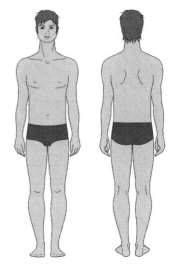

Notes

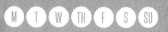
	Time	Blood Sugar	Carbs	Insulin	Notes
Breakfast					
Snack					
Lunch					
Snack					
Dinner					
Bedtime					
Night					

Shot Location

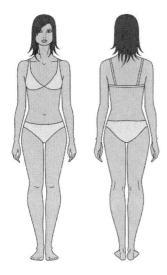
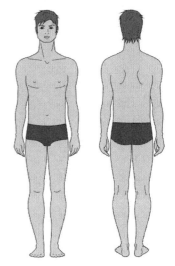

Notes

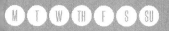

M T W TH F S SU

Date: /   /

	Time	Blood Sugar	Carbs	Insulin	Notes
Breakfast					
Snack					
Lunch					
Snack					
Dinner					
Bedtime					
Night					

Shot Location

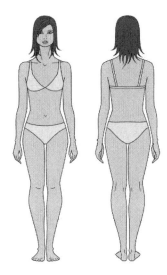

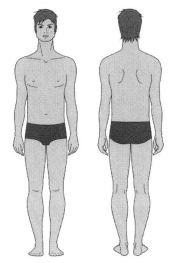

Notes

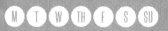
	Time	Blood Sugar	Carbs	Insulin	Notes
Breakfast					
Snack					
Lunch					
Snack					
Dinner					
Bedtime					
Night					

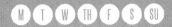

Shot Location

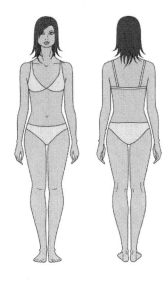 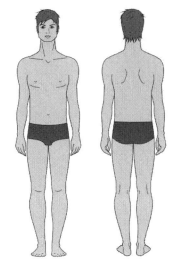

Notes

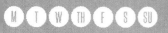
	Time	Blood Sugar	Carbs	Insulin	Notes
Breakfast					
Snack					
Lunch					
Snack					
Dinner					
Bedtime					
Night					

Shot Location

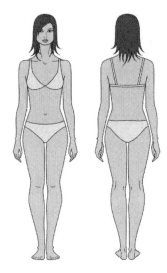 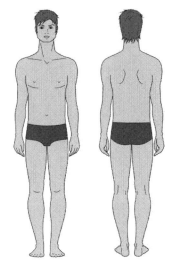

Notes

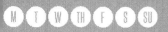
	Time	Blood Sugar	Carbs	Insulin	Notes
Breakfast					
Snack					
Lunch					
Snack					
Dinner					
Bedtime					
Night					

Shot Location

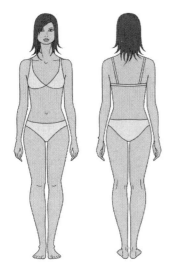

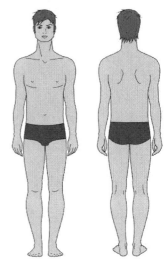

Notes

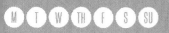

Date: / /

	Time	Blood Sugar	Carbs	Insulin	Notes
Breakfast					
Snack					
Lunch					
Snack					
Dinner					
Bedtime					
Night					

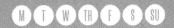
Shot Location

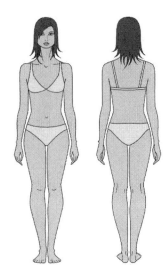

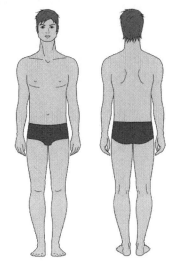

Notes

	Time	Blood Sugar	Carbs	Insulin	Notes
Breakfast					
Snack					
Lunch					
Snack					
Dinner					
Bedtime					
Night					

Shot Location

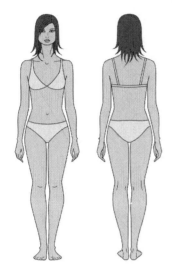

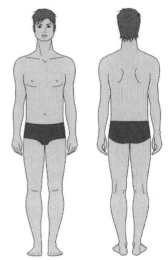

Notes

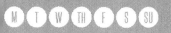

Date: /   /

	Time	Blood Sugar	Carbs	Insulin	Notes
Breakfast					
Snack					
Lunch					
Snack					
Dinner					
Bedtime					
Night					

Shot Location

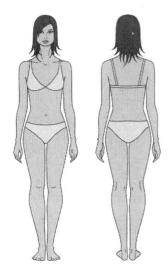

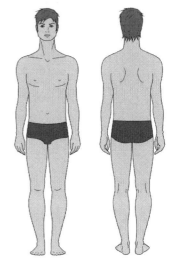

Notes

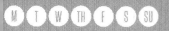

Date: /   /

	Time	Blood Sugar	Carbs	Insulin	Notes
Breakfast					
Snack					
Lunch					
Snack					
Dinner					
Bedtime					
Night					

Shot Location

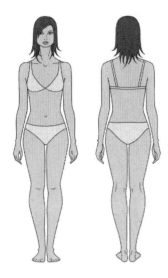

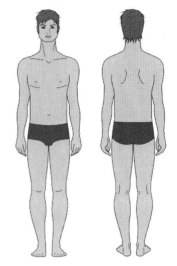

Notes

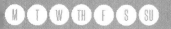
	Time	Blood Sugar	Carbs	Insulin	Notes
Breakfast					
Snack					
Lunch					
Snack					
Dinner					
Bedtime					
Night					

Shot Location

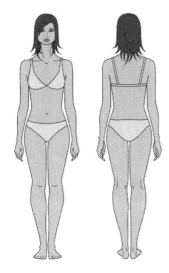
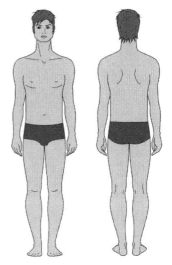

Notes

	Time	Blood Sugar	Carbs	Insulin	Notes
Breakfast					
Snack					
Lunch					
Snack					
Dinner					
Bedtime					
Night					

Shot Location

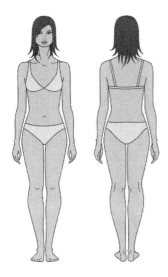

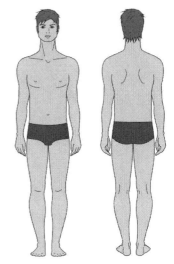

Notes

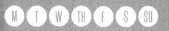

	Time	Blood Sugar	Carbs	Insulin	Notes
Breakfast					
Snack					
Lunch					
Snack					
Dinner					
Bedtime					
Night					

Shot Location

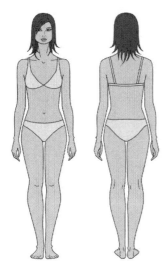

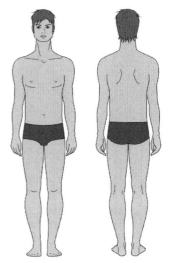

Notes

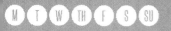

	Time	Blood Sugar	Carbs	Insulin	Notes
Breakfast					
Snack					
Lunch					
Snack					
Dinner					
Bedtime					
Night					

Shot Location

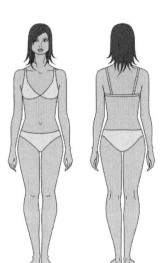
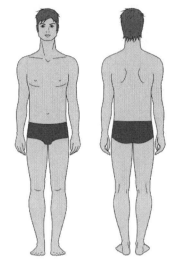

Notes

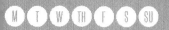

M T W TH F S SU

Date: / /

	Time	Blood Sugar	Carbs	Insulin	Notes
Breakfast					
Snack					
Lunch					
Snack					
Dinner					
Bedtime					
Night					

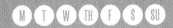
Shot Location

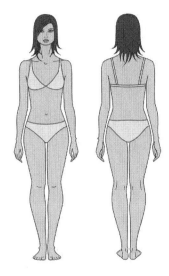 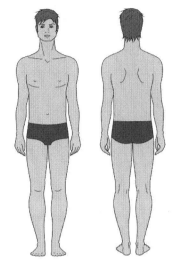

Notes

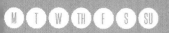
	Time	Blood Sugar	Carbs	Insulin	Notes
Breakfast					
Snack					
Lunch					
Snack					
Dinner					
Bedtime					
Night					

Shot Location

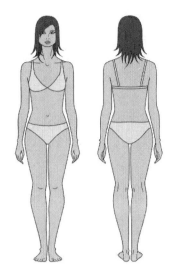

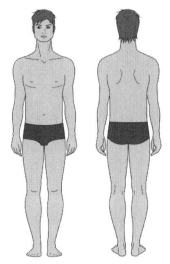

Notes

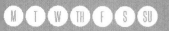

	Time	Blood Sugar	Carbs	Insulin	Notes
Breakfast					
Snack					
Lunch					
Snack					
Dinner					
Bedtime					
Night					

Shot Location

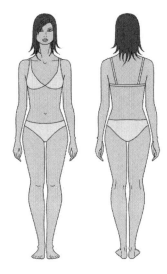 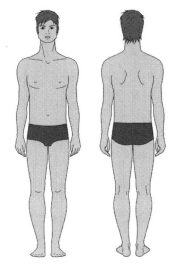

Notes

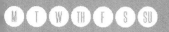
	Time	Blood Sugar	Carbs	Insulin	Notes
Breakfast					
Snack					
Lunch					
Snack					
Dinner					
Bedtime					
Night					

Shot Location

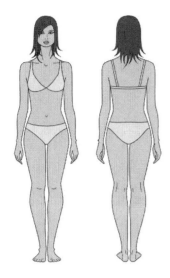

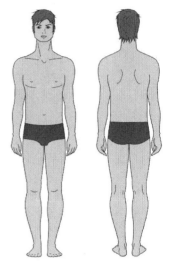

Notes

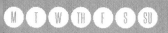

Date: / /

	Time	Blood Sugar	Carbs	Insulin	Notes
Breakfast					
Snack					
Lunch					
Snack					
Dinner					
Bedtime					
Night					

Shot Location

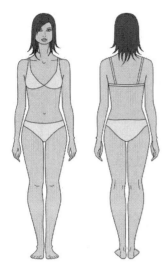
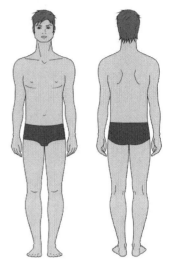

Notes

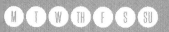

	Time	Blood Sugar	Carbs	Insulin	Notes
Breakfast					
Snack					
Lunch					
Snack					
Dinner					
Bedtime					
Night					

Shot Location

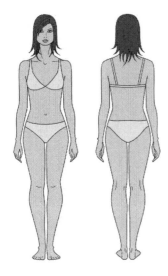

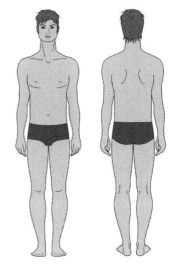

Notes

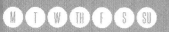

Date: / /

	Time	Blood Sugar	Carbs	Insulin	Notes
Breakfast					
Snack					
Lunch					
Snack					
Dinner					
Bedtime					
Night					

Shot Location

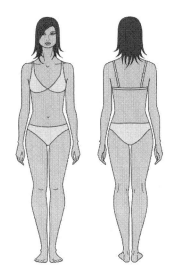
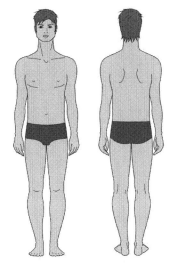

Notes

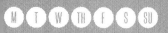

Date: / /

	Time	Blood Sugar	Carbs	Insulin	Notes
Breakfast					
Snack					
Lunch					
Snack					
Dinner					
Bedtime					
Night					

Shot Location

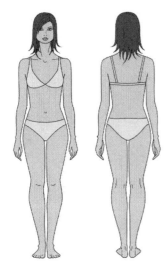

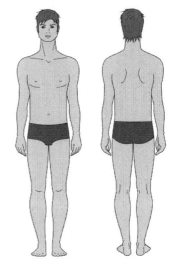

Notes

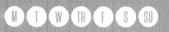

Date: /   /

	Time	Blood Sugar	Carbs	Insulin	Notes
Breakfast					
Snack					
Lunch					
Snack					
Dinner					
Bedtime					
Night					

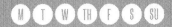
Shot Location

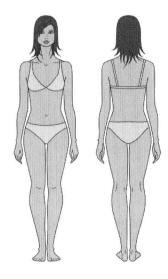 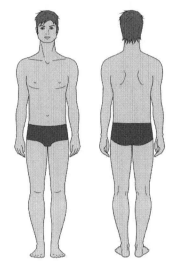

Notes

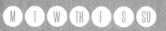
	Time	Blood Sugar	Carbs	Insulin	Notes
Breakfast					
Snack					
Lunch					
Snack					
Dinner					
Bedtime					
Night					

Shot Location

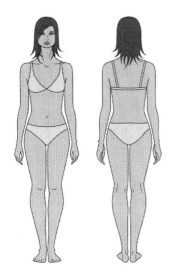

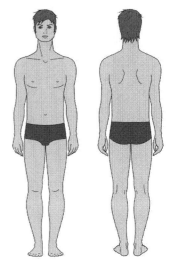

Notes

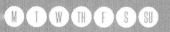

Date: / /

	Time	Blood Sugar	Carbs	Insulin	Notes
Breakfast					
Snack					
Lunch					
Snack					
Dinner					
Bedtime					
Night					

Shot Location

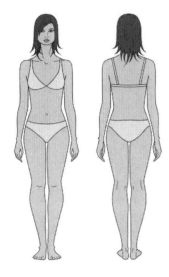

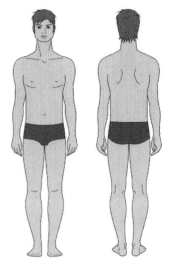

Notes

	Time	Blood Sugar	Carbs	Insulin	Notes
Breakfast					
Snack					
Lunch					
Snack					
Dinner					
Bedtime					
Night					

Shot Location

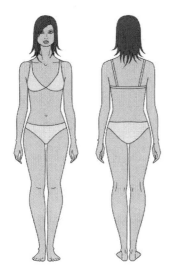
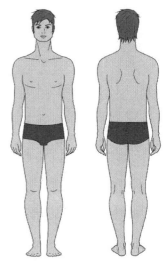

Notes

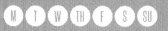

	Time	Blood Sugar	Carbs	Insulin	Notes
Breakfast					
Snack					
Lunch					
Snack					
Dinner					
Bedtime					
Night					

Shot Location

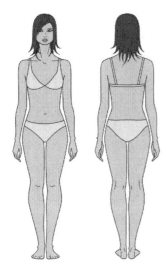 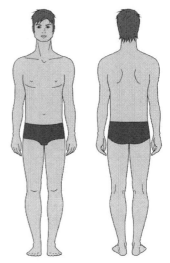

Notes

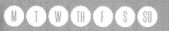
	Time	Blood Sugar	Carbs	Insulin	Notes
Breakfast					
Snack					
Lunch					
Snack					
Dinner					
Bedtime					
Night					

Shot Location

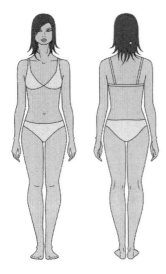

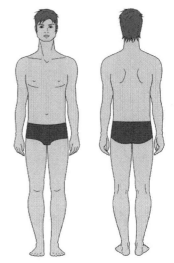

Notes

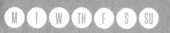
	Time	Blood Sugar	Carbs	Insulin	Notes
Breakfast					
Snack					
Lunch					
Snack					
Dinner					
Bedtime					
Night					

Shot Location

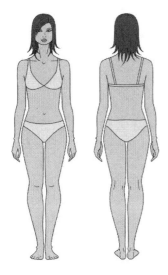
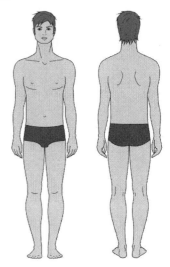

Notes

	Time	Blood Sugar	Carbs	Insulin	Notes
Breakfast					
Snack					
Lunch					
Snack					
Dinner					
Bedtime					
Night					

Shot Location

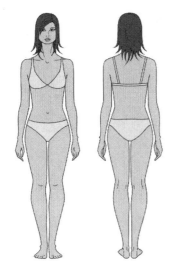
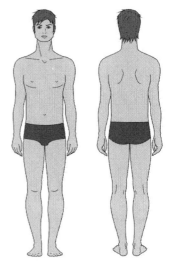

Notes

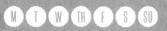

Date: / /

	Time	Blood Sugar	Carbs	Insulin	Notes
Breakfast					
Snack					
Lunch					
Snack					
Dinner					
Bedtime					
Night					

Shot Location

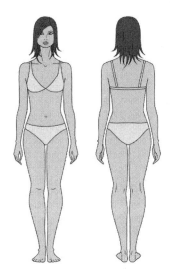

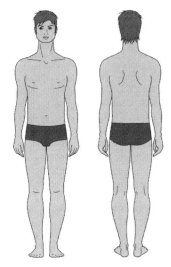

Notes

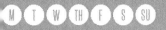

	Time	Blood Sugar	Carbs	Insulin	Notes
Breakfast					
Snack					
Lunch					
Snack					
Dinner					
Bedtime					
Night					

Shot Location

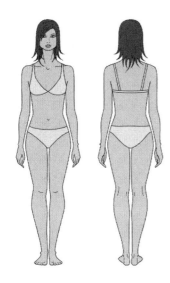

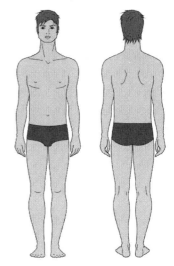

Notes

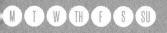
	Time	Blood Sugar	Carbs	Insulin	Notes
Breakfast					
Snack					
Lunch					
Snack					
Dinner					
Bedtime					
Night					

Shot Location

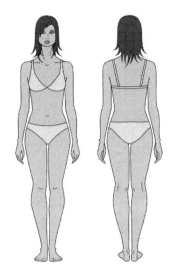

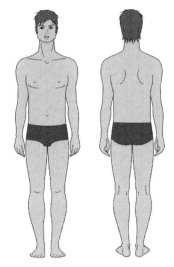

Notes

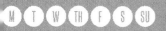

Date: /   /

	Time	Blood Sugar	Carbs	Insulin	Notes
Breakfast					
Snack					
Lunch					
Snack					
Dinner					
Bedtime					
Night					

Shot Location

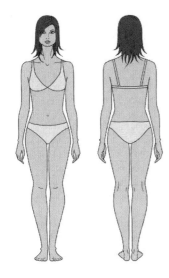

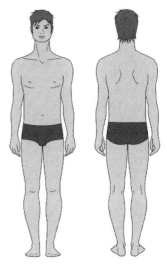

Notes

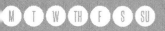

Date: /   /

	Time	Blood Sugar	Carbs	Insulin	Notes
Breakfast					
Snack					
Lunch					
Snack					
Dinner					
Bedtime					
Night					

Shot Location

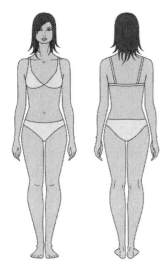

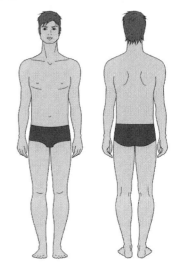

Notes

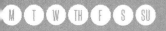

M T W TH F S SU

Date: / /

	Time	Blood Sugar	Carbs	Insulin	Notes
Breakfast					
Snack					
Lunch					
Snack					
Dinner					
Bedtime					
Night					

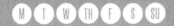
Shot Location

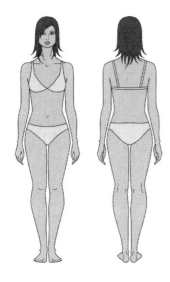 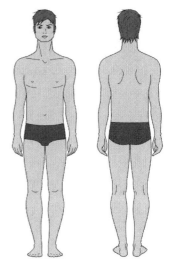

Notes

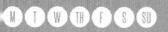
	Time	Blood Sugar	Carbs	Insulin	Notes
Breakfast					
Snack					
Lunch					
Snack					
Dinner					
Bedtime					
Night					

Shot Location

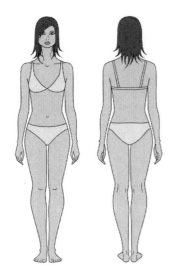

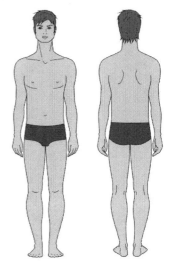

Notes

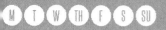
	Time	Blood Sugar	Carbs	Insulin	Notes
Breakfast					
Snack					
Lunch					
Snack					
Dinner					
Bedtime					
Night					

Shot Location

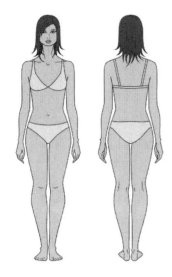 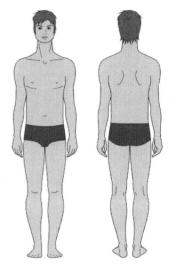

Notes

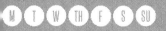

Date: / /

	Time	Blood Sugar	Carbs	Insulin	Notes
Breakfast					
Snack					
Lunch					
Snack					
Dinner					
Bedtime					
Night					

Shot Location

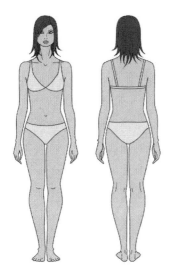

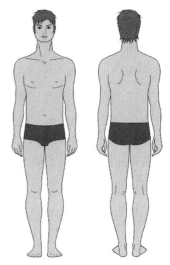

Notes

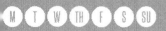
	Time	Blood Sugar	Carbs	Insulin	Notes
Breakfast					
Snack					
Lunch					
Snack					
Dinner					
Bedtime					
Night					

Shot Location

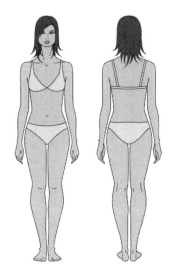 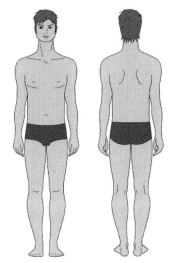

Notes

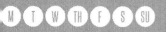

	Time	Blood Sugar	Carbs	Insulin	Notes
Breakfast					
Snack					
Lunch					
Snack					
Dinner					
Bedtime					
Night					

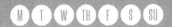

Shot Location

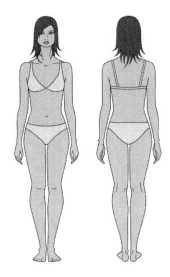 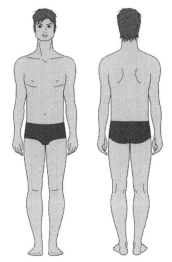

Notes

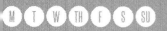

M T W TH F S SU

Date: / /

	Time	Blood Sugar	Carbs	Insulin	Notes
Breakfast					
Snack					
Lunch					
Snack					
Dinner					
Bedtime					
Night					

Shot Location

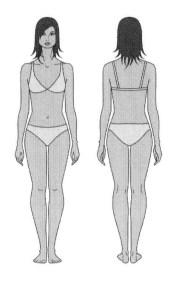
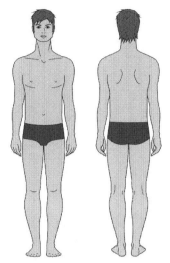

Notes

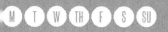
	Time	Blood Sugar	Carbs	Insulin	Notes
Breakfast					
Snack					
Lunch					
Snack					
Dinner					
Bedtime					
Night					

Shot Location

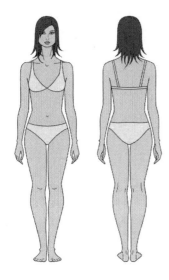 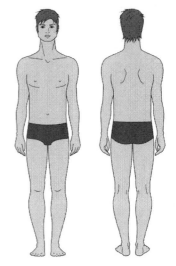

Notes

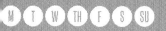
	Time	Blood Sugar	Carbs	Insulin	Notes
Breakfast					
Snack					
Lunch					
Snack					
Dinner					
Bedtime					
Night					

Shot Location

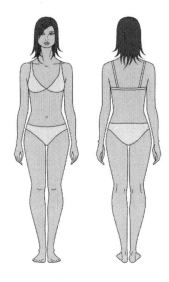

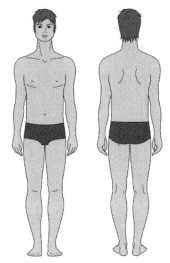

Notes

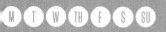

M T W TH F S SU

Date: / /

	Time	Blood Sugar	Carbs	Insulin	Notes
Breakfast					
Snack					
Lunch					
Snack					
Dinner					
Bedtime					
Night					

Shot Location

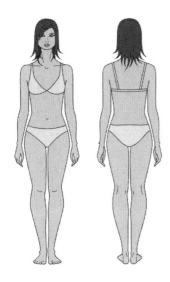 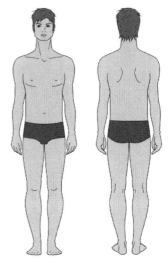

Notes

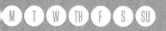
	Time	Blood Sugar	Carbs	Insulin	Notes
Breakfast					
Snack					
Lunch					
Snack					
Dinner					
Bedtime					
Night					

Shot Location

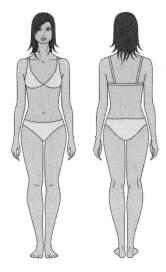
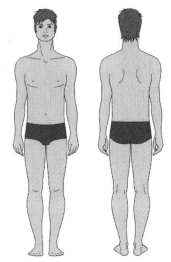

Notes

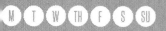
	Time	Blood Sugar	Carbs	Insulin	Notes
Breakfast					
Snack					
Lunch					
Snack					
Dinner					
Bedtime					
Night					

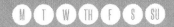

Shot Location

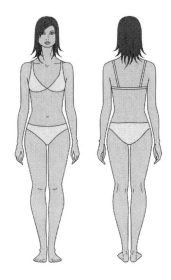

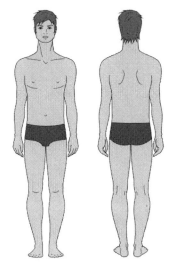

Notes

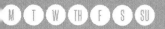
	Time	Blood Sugar	Carbs	Insulin	Notes
Breakfast					
Snack					
Lunch					
Snack					
Dinner					
Bedtime					
Night					

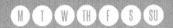

Shot Location

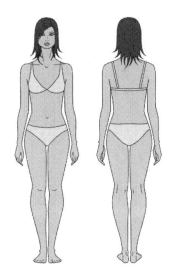

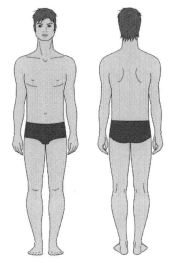

Notes

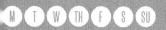
	Time	Blood Sugar	Carbs	Insulin	Notes
Breakfast					
Snack					
Lunch					
Snack					
Dinner					
Bedtime					
Night					

Shot Location

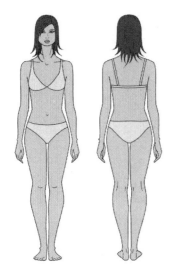

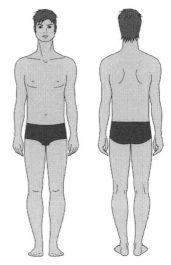

Notes

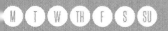

M T W TH F S SU

Date: / /

	Time	Blood Sugar	Carbs	Insulin	Notes
Breakfast					
Snack					
Lunch					
Snack					
Dinner					
Bedtime					
Night					

Shot Location

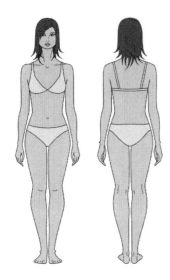 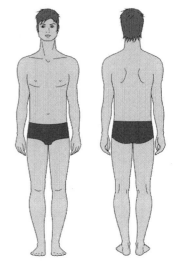

Notes

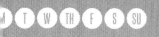
	Time	Blood Sugar	Carbs	Insulin	Notes
Breakfast					
Snack					
Lunch					
Snack					
Dinner					
Bedtime					
Night					

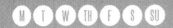

Shot Location

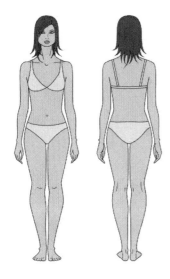

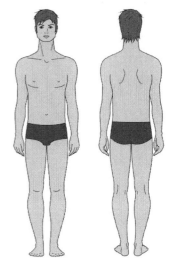

Notes

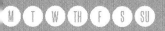

M T W TH F S SU

Date: /   /

	Time	Blood Sugar	Carbs	Insulin	Notes
Breakfast					
Snack					
Lunch					
Snack					
Dinner					
Bedtime					
Night					

Shot Location

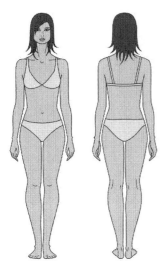
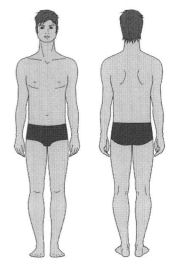

Notes

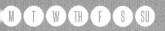

	Time	Blood Sugar	Carbs	Insulin	Notes
Breakfast					
Snack					
Lunch					
Snack					
Dinner					
Bedtime					
Night					

Shot Location

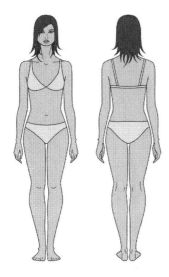

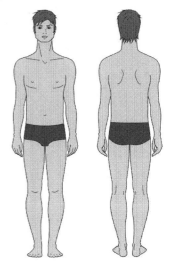

Notes

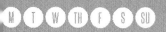

	Time	Blood Sugar	Carbs	Insulin	Notes
Breakfast					
Snack					
Lunch					
Snack					
Dinner					
Bedtime					
Night					

Shot Location

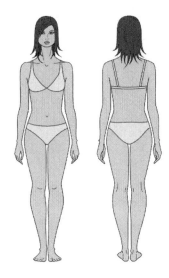

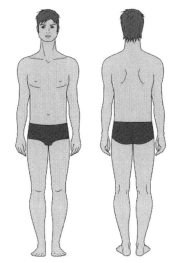

Notes

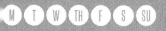

	Time	Blood Sugar	Carbs	Insulin	Notes
Breakfast					
Snack					
Lunch					
Snack					
Dinner					
Bedtime					
Night					

Shot Location

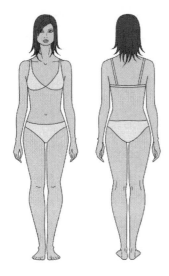 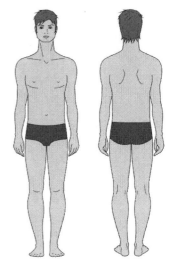

Notes

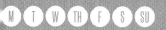

	Time	Blood Sugar	Carbs	Insulin	Notes
Breakfast					
Snack					
Lunch					
Snack					
Dinner					
Bedtime					
Night					

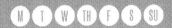
Shot Location

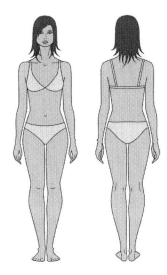

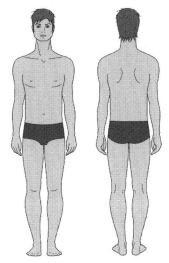

Notes

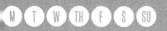

Date: /   /

	Time	Blood Sugar	Carbs	Insulin	Notes
Breakfast					
Snack					
Lunch					
Snack					
Dinner					
Bedtime					
Night					

Shot Location

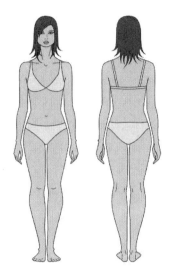

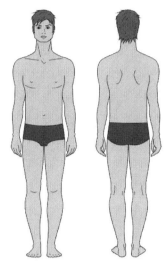

Notes

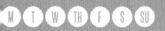
	Time	Blood Sugar	Carbs	Insulin	Notes
Breakfast					
Snack					
Lunch					
Snack					
Dinner					
Bedtime					
Night					

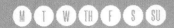

Shot Location

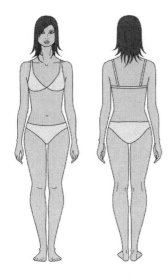

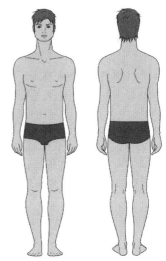

Notes

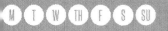

M T W TH F S SU

Date: / /

	Time	Blood Sugar	Carbs	Insulin	Notes
Breakfast					
Snack					
Lunch					
Snack					
Dinner					
Bedtime					
Night					

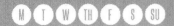

Shot Location

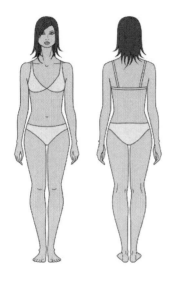

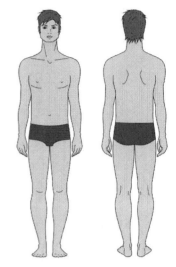

Notes

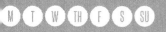
	Time	Blood Sugar	Carbs	Insulin	Notes
Breakfast					
Snack					
Lunch					
Snack					
Dinner					
Bedtime					
Night					

Shot Location

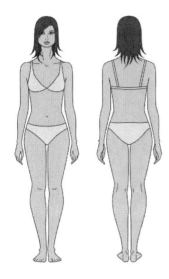 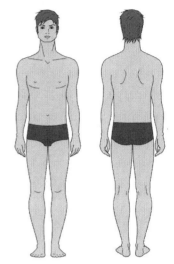

Notes

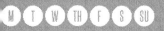

	Time	Blood Sugar	Carbs	Insulin	Notes
Breakfast					
Snack					
Lunch					
Snack					
Dinner					
Bedtime					
Night					

Shot Location

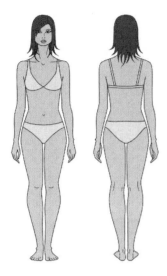
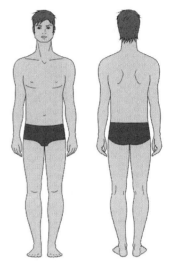

Notes

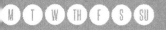
	Time	Blood Sugar	Carbs	Insulin	Notes
Breakfast					
Snack					
Lunch					
Snack					
Dinner					
Bedtime					
Night					

Shot Location

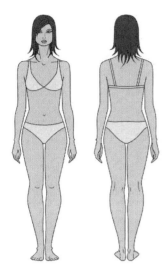

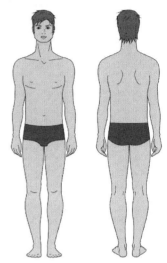

Notes

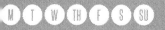
	Time	Blood Sugar	Carbs	Insulin	Notes
Breakfast					
Snack					
Lunch					
Snack					
Dinner					
Bedtime					
Night					

Shot Location

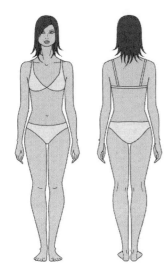

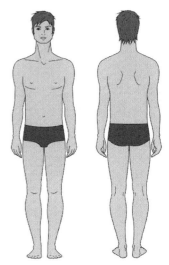

Notes

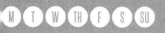

	Time	Blood Sugar	Carbs	Insulin	Notes
Breakfast					
Snack					
Lunch					
Snack					
Dinner					
Bedtime					
Night					

Shot Location

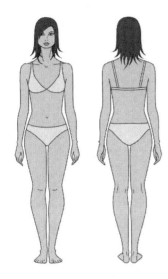 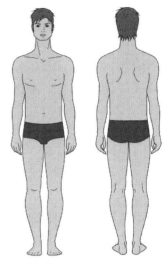

Notes

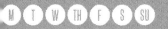

M T W TH F S SU

Date: / /

	Time	Blood Sugar	Carbs	Insulin	Notes
Breakfast					
Snack					
Lunch					
Snack					
Dinner					
Bedtime					
Night					

Shot Location

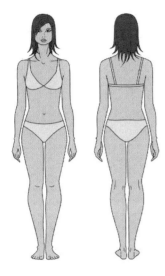 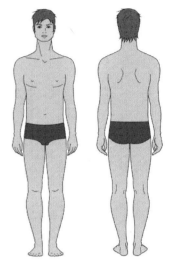

Notes

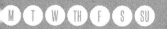

Date: / /

	Time	Blood Sugar	Carbs	Insulin	Notes
Breakfast					
Snack					
Lunch					
Snack					
Dinner					
Bedtime					
Night					

Shot Location

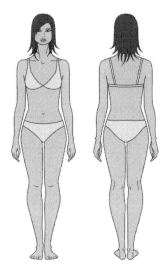

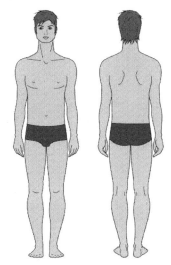

Notes

	Time	Blood Sugar	Carbs	Insulin	Notes
Breakfast					
Snack					
Lunch					
Snack					
Dinner					
Bedtime					
Night					

Shot Location

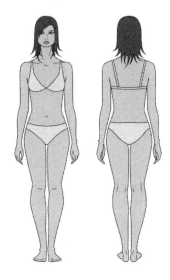
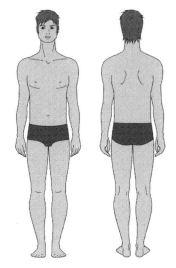

Notes

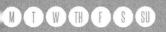
	Time	Blood Sugar	Carbs	Insulin	Notes
Breakfast					
Snack					
Lunch					
Snack					
Dinner					
Bedtime					
Night					

Shot Location

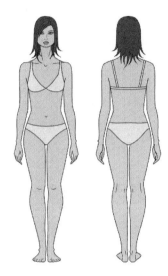
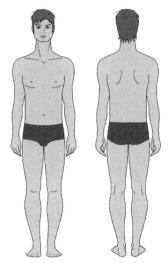

Notes

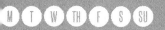

M T W TH F S SU

Date: / /

	Time	Blood Sugar	Carbs	Insulin	Notes
Breakfast					
Snack					
Lunch					
Snack					
Dinner					
Bedtime					
Night					

Shot Location

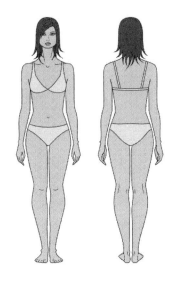

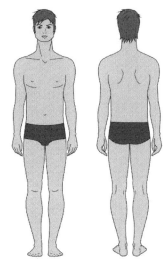

Notes

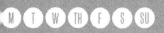

M T W TH F S SU

Date: / /

	Time	Blood Sugar	Carbs	Insulin	Notes
Breakfast					
Snack					
Lunch					
Snack					
Dinner					
Bedtime					
Night					

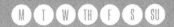
Shot Location

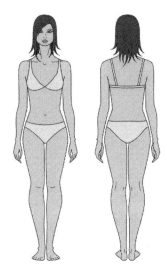

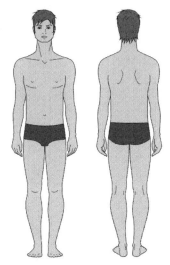

Notes

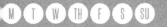
	Time	Blood Sugar	Carbs	Insulin	Notes
Breakfast					
Snack					
Lunch					
Snack					
Dinner					
Bedtime					
Night					

Shot Location

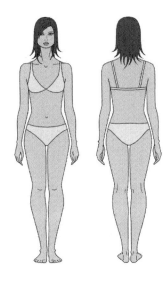

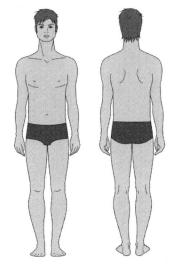

Notes

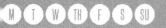
	Time	Blood Sugar	Carbs	Insulin	Notes
Breakfast					
Snack					
Lunch					
Snack					
Dinner					
Bedtime					
Night					

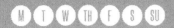

Shot Location

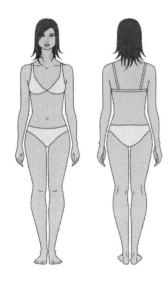

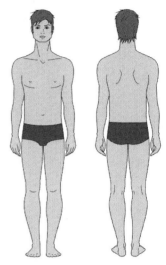

Notes

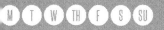
	Time	Blood Sugar	Carbs	Insulin	Notes
Breakfast					
Snack					
Lunch					
Snack					
Dinner					
Bedtime					
Night					

Made in the USA
Middletown, DE
29 April 2021